Faith Of One Mustard Seed

My 18-Year Journey to Motherhood While Battling PCOS

TAMEKA L. CHAPMAN

ISBN: 1983654329
ISBN-13: 978-1983654329

DEDICATION

To my son, Aspen Baylor.
You are mommy's sunshine and my moon!
You are my WHY.

To my husband, Deone,
For being my biggest supporter and staying by my side
through it all. You have loved me, flaws and all.

To God,
For blessing me with the strength to endure the wait.

To my fellow PCOS cysters,
I pray that you remain hopeful for your heart's desire of
having children of your own.

TABLE OF CONTENTS

ACKNOWLEDGMENTS

First, giving honor to God, who is the head of my life. Thank you for the life that You have given me. Because of the many tests that You've administered and gotten me through, I now have the greatest testimony to share with the world.

To both of my grandmothers, Gussie Lee and Ora Lee (*Rest In Heaven, Madear*), you both have inspired me in different ways that has allowed me to be the woman I am today. I will love you forever.

To my family, Daddy, Ma, Aunt Cynt and my Heavenly Angels Aunt Pearl and Mommy Sylvia, thank you for always having an open ear and heart, even during the times that I may not have been tuned in to your wisdom.

To my Aunt Salane, at 13 years old, you prayed for me and over me and I have always kept that prayer close to me. In your prayer, you said that everything I touched would "turn to gold." I have lived my life believing just that and I have now given birth to "The Golden Child", your great-nephew Aspen Baylor.

To my Sister, Alicia, I thank God for blessing me with you. You are my little gem of love! Thank you for the constant laughter and talks. They mean so much to me.

To my Brothers, JJ and Daryl, thank you for your never-ending sibling love and side-bursting laughter. You are the best & I love you!

To the Best Big Sisters in the world, Pam and Shawn, your great talks and listening ears have been a total blessing to me during these past 5 years. I'm thankful for the honesty, frankness, and loyalty you possess. I love you dearly.

To the Best Baby Shower Hosts EVER. Pam, Shawn, Hemma, Brittany, Era, and Donna. You don't know how much it meant to me to know that you great ladies wanted to do something so special for me and my little blessing. I totally appreciate the love you have shown. You are the BEST!

To my family and friends that have been my morning laughter, my mid-week smile, and evening talks. I'm lucky to have so many great people in my life.

To Kenny Jones for being my last and biggest inspiration of 2017. Thank you, my brother, for allowing others in your life in the most open & honest way. I'm proud to be called a #ComebackKid. You Are Awesome!

To my son, Aspen Baylor Chapman.
Thank you for being my constant reminder that God Is Real.

FOREWORD

There are many times throughout a woman's life when she may feel depressed, discouraged, and disheartened. Getting passed over for a promotion, ending a marriage, and even having a major argument with a close girlfriend are life events that could spark these types of emotions. Although these life events can create emotional triggers for a woman, the loss of an unborn child during pregnancy or the disappointment that comes from numerous unsuccessful rounds of IVF fertility treatments can send a woman into an emotional abyss that seemingly has no end in sight.

It is during these dark times that she must lean on her faith and reaffirm in her spirit that if she holds on to just a tiny bit of faith, God will carry her through her darkest moments into the marvelous light of unspeakable joy. I am reminded of God's faithfulness to us in Tameka L. Chapman's book *Faith of One Mustard Seed: My 18-Year Journey to Motherhood While Battling PCOS*. The book is a must read for any woman who is going through something and feels like she is all alone.

From the first time I met Tameka, I knew there was something very special about her. She had a quiet unassuming presence that illuminated the room. I had no idea that Tameka had been trying to have a baby with no success. I assumed that she didn't want any children or that she and her husband were intentionally waiting to have children. Her secret suffering went unnoticed because she did such a good job of hiding her pain.

Tameka's infectious personality made it easy to talk to her. She was always bubbly and full of laughter. How could someone who was so fun to be around be so miserable inside? This is a question I asked myself over and over again as I read the book. We connected early on because we both had fertility issues in common. She shared her story with me and I shared my story with her. We have laughed, cried, and even prayed together.

The book takes the reader on a rollercoaster of emotions that every woman who has ever had fertility issues can relate to. The reader will experience the highs and lows of trying to conceive a child for eighteen long years. Any woman who reads this book will know that her darkest moments can become the most joyous moments of her life.

I am inspired by Tameka's story and I know that you will be inspired too. Whenever you feel like you want to give up on a dream, desire, or goal that God told you would happen, remember to hold onto that dream with the faith of a mustard seed, and your dreams will come to fruition.

SHAWN JACKSON WILSON

1 IT WAS ALL A DREAM

Imagine me, loving what I see when the mirror looks at me 'cause I, I imagine me in a place of no insecurities and I'm finally happy 'cause I imagine me. ~ Imagine Me, Kirk Franklin

For as long as I can remember, I've always wanted to be a mother. I dreamed of hearing a little boy saying mama, mommy or mom while lovingly looking at me. I dreamed of how I would gaze into my little one's eyes and see the pure innocence he'd possess. I dreamed of how I'd raise him and show him the world. I dreamed of how he'd be a successful man because of all the love, tough love and examples that I would ensure he would be shown. It was all a dream and I couldn't wait for it to happen.

Although it was my dream, I knew it would become my reality, but I also knew that I had to make sure that my life was stable in every way before I would be ready to care for my precious child.

Like many, I've had situations and circumstances to happen in life that made me start to question everything and everybody, including God, at times. Death even came knocking on my door three times throughout the past 18 years. And each time it knocked, God stepped in to say, "Not Now", and spared my life. At one point, I didn't feel that I was worthy of living and felt all kinds of ways that no one should ever feel about themselves. I had allowed depression to come in and take residence in my mentality and didn't even realize it. I was spinning out of control and I didn't want to talk to anybody about it.

Have you ever felt alone even in the midst of people that loved you? That was me. Instead of talking to any of my family or friends, I decided *for them* that they wouldn't understand what I was going through. I felt it was better to keep things to myself, which was, as I now realize, not the best decision to make. Keeping my feelings inside and not properly dealing with them only lead to catastrophe, but I didn't know that I had *real* issues that I needed to address. I felt as if it was normal to feel the way I felt, disappointed and sad, due to all that I was going through to create my own family.

As I started to work on the issues that I knew that I had, each time I thought I was ready, I would find another area of my life that needed adjusting.

I've worked long and hard to be the person that I am today. Let me tell you, I absolutely love who I am today! I've worked hard to get back to my faith and believing everything that God promised me, He'd give me. Someone once told me that they wished that they had half of the courage that I exude. What? I simply told them that when you have the faith the size of only ONE mustard seed, you can achieve anything in life that you desire. Just be sure to remember that everything comes to your life at its predetermined time by God.

I hope that you allow my journey to serve as an inspiration for you to continue having faith or to start having faith. Believe that everything your heart desires can be realized. What was once a dream for me has now turned into my reality, all because I kept the faith.

I am a living testimony!

And Jesus said unto them, Because of your unbelief: for verily I say unto you, If ye have faith as a grain of mustard seed, ye shall say unto this mountain, Remove hence to yonder place; and it shall remove; and nothing shall be impossible unto you.

Matthew 17:20 Bible, King James Version

2 WHAT MARRIAGE MEANT TO ME

Fortunate to have you girl. I'm so glad you're in my world. Just as sure as the sky is blue. I bless the day that I found you. ~ Fortunate, Maxwell

In late November of 1998, I met a man who I was not looking to meet at that time in my life. I've always believed that the man should pursue the woman, so if that didn't happen anytime soon, I was fine with waiting. When he approached me, my guard was up because I had met many bad characters who weren't good for me.

This man made me laugh. He would have me laughing so hard that I'd be in tears with aching sides.

This man was protective. Some (*me*) would call him overbearing, at times, but who wouldn't want a knight in shiny armor?

This man was patient. He allowed our friendship to blossom without any demands for a title.

This man was caring. He wasn't embarrassed to hang out with me or check on me when I wasn't feeling well.

This man made me feel comfortable in being myself. I felt that I could talk to him and tell him everything. We had natural chemistry and it felt great to be in his presence.

This was a real man and, I believed, that this was the man that God sent to me.

Even though I wasn't looking for a relationship, I knew he was the ONE. He possessed and showed all the great qualities that a man should possess. He treated me like his Queen and had no problem letting others know that I was his "old lady." This is a southern term for your wife/girlfriend, after being together for a very long time. To me, he knew that I was the one for him too even though we had never discussed it.

After dating for three and a half months, this man decided to let the world know that I was the ONE for him too. On Monday, February 8, 1999, he popped the question. On Tuesday, February 9, 1999, we went ring shopping, and later, we went to the courthouse to register to be wedded. We were married 3 days later, on Friday, February 12, 1999.

WOW!!! That was one of the most exciting days of my life even though I hadn't told my family that I was in a serious relationship or that I was getting married. Of course, I called them right after and let them know. There was a bit of disbelief, at first, but as I knew my family, they embraced my husband and our relationship because I was genuinely happy.

To me, marriage meant the beginning of a new and exciting chapter in my life. It meant that I was able to have this man as my protector, best friend, and soulmate for the rest of our lives. I truly believe in 'til death do us part, so he was now stuck with me, flaws and all.

Marriage meant that I was now a full-grown woman and no longer the young lady that needed to call home each time something happened. I now had to handle our new life situations and circumstances with my husband.

Marriage meant that we were able to do and go as we desired, as a couple. While in our honeymoon phase, we would do impromptu road trips, go to the movies, learn about each other's living style and families (since we didn't live with each other prior to getting married). We purchased and decorated our first home, found more similarities in each other, and learned to love each other even more.

Marriage meant that I'd have someone to laugh at my corny jokes and not give me the side-eye. It meant that we could stay in our pajamas and lounge around the house ALL DAY, if we desired.

Marriage meant that he accepted me for who I am truly was, flaws and all. Flaws that I knew about and the flaws that were invisible.

Marriage meant that I could buy everything that said, "His & Hers" or "Mr. & Mrs.", and it would really mean something to us.

Marriage meant that we could walk around the house in our robes acting as if we were King & Queen while listening to Maxwell serenade us for as long as we wanted. It also meant making fun of each other and being able to laugh about it.

Ultimately, to me, marriage meant that we'd be able to start the family that I always knew I wanted. I wanted to have children, three children to be exact, so that I could teach them everything they would need to know to survive in this crazy world. They would have each other when the world turned cold and would be pillars of support for each other. I would give them all the love that I possessed. I wanted to watch them grow up, say their first words, take their first steps, and smile for the first time. I was so excited that we were about to start our family.

If I knew then what I know now.

Little did we know or imagine the many struggles and hardships we'd face in our quest to have a family of our own.

3 WHY NOT ME?

I, I can't even turn on the phone without being reminded of the lie that I am alone and broken, unsuccessful. I, I can't always talk to my friends 'cause they've got expectations that I may or may not be living up to. I really need to rid myself of the pressure, pressure, pressure to be someone else that the world has made. Jesus take from me all the pressure, pressure, pressure to be someone that you did not create. ~ Pressure, Jonathan McReynolds

In 2000, and after trying to start our family for one whole year, it seemed as if it would never happen. Because my husband was still serving in the military, I felt that it was OK to continue to try, but not push it too hard because I didn't believe that I was created to be a single mother. His career would take him away from home for many months at a time, sometimes seven to eight months out of the year. Talk about a long-distance relationship!

Every month when he was home, we'd try and, every month, the test results were negative. This was the start of my heart breaking. Each month, my heart would break a little more. It felt as if I could feel a piece of my heart chipping away, bit by bit, and falling into an abyss of nothingness. I started to feel empty.

I can, officially, say that this was the beginning of my sadness, my self-sabotaging behavior, my internal hatred, my depression, my desire to be left alone, and my desire to crawl in a dark hole and hide from all women and their beautiful children. This was the start of it all becoming too much for me to handle. Feeling ashamed and insecure about my womanhood stopped me from reaching out to any of my friends or family for support. I made the decision *for* them that they wouldn't understand.

As much as I loved to smile, my true smile was hidden by my constant disappointment. The smile that I showed hid my fears, doubts, self-consciousness, sadness and depression. My smile hid my true self. I was beginning to tune the world out and I was beginning to not be my authentic self. I would push away anyone that tried to be a friend. I don't even think I could be that great of a friend because of all the internal noise that was holding my mentality in captivity.

Here I was, a 21-year-old woman with a heart of gold and a silent struggle within. I became shameful of my struggle. I didn't allow my family and friends to relate and show me the support that I needed. Most of them already had kids. How can they understand what I was going through? I started hating Mother's Day and started resenting any mother who I felt wasn't being the greatest mom to their kids. I would see a child with what I perceived as improper clothing and I would have something to say about her parenting. I became so judgmental! It was wrong, and I was hurting.

The year 2000 was the beginning of my downfall season that lasted for the next 15 years. I became a bit more withdrawn, all while wearing a smile. I knew it had gotten worse because I asked my husband, my soulmate, and best friend, if he wanted to divorce me so that he could find someone to give him the children I knew he wanted in his life. As the true man that was placed on this earth for me, he wasn't trying to hear any of that nonsense. He was set on finding a solution so that we could start our own beautiful family. Was I glad that he chose to stay with me? Absolutely. Did it help with how I was feeling? Absolutely not.

I was raised with the understanding that we never question God because He is God Almighty, but I needed answers and nobody on this earth could provide them. I began thinking it was OK to question God and His plan for my life. Was I not living right? Was I not created to be a mother? Was I not good enough to have the title of mother? Did He not trust me to care for a child? What was wrong with me? Was there something in my past for which I needed to repent to receive my blessings? I didn't know what more to do or what more for which to pray.

That last question made me start a complete review of my entire life. In doing so, I opened wounds that had never been healed, and I felt as if I released internal demons from my past that I had chosen to not face. As a child, I didn't know how to deal with those feelings or demons and, because I didn't want to be seen as crazy, I kept it all inside. It was all bottled up, and over the course of my life, all of it would be released in ways that I couldn't even imagine.

Facing My Past Was Hard

I began thinking back to my childhood, as far back as I could remember. I started thinking of actions that may not have been the right thing to do. I remembered how I would sometimes roll my eyes at the adults because they were saying things that I didn't want to hear. I asked God for forgiveness. I remembered the stupid sibling fights and how they should have never happened. I asked God for forgiveness. I remembered feeling alone and taking my despair out on anyone that I could. I asked God for forgiveness. I remembered how I would say (*to myself*) that I hated my life. I asked God for forgiveness. I remembered how I would feel like the oddball and I had thoughts of not wanting to be live anymore. I asked God for forgiveness. I remembered using foul language to those who didn't deserve it. I asked God for forgiveness. I remembered being sexually assaulted. Although this wasn't my wrong, I asked God for forgiveness for the feelings that I was still holding on to. I remembered pulling away from loved ones, trying to make a point by hurting them. I asked God for forgiveness. I remembered getting upset with my husband when he was trying his best to understand. I asked God for forgiveness.

This was not a one-day or two-day conversation with God. These memories came to me over time. I could see the memories as though they were happening all over again, in living color. I would see my wrongs; I would see what I should have done differently, and I would ask God for forgiveness.

This year, I started doubting everything and everyone around me. Doubting everyone was my way of giving myself a reason to add distance. I thought this was the answer and the best way to deal, but in truth, it was the worst. I really enjoyed talking to everyone and pulling away only made me sadder. I was alienating myself from people that knew me and would support me the best way they knew how, if I would only give them the chance. My decision to suffer alone and in silence was unfair to me and them.

Fertility Specialist 1

Going into 2001, I had had enough! I could no longer sit back and wait. After all, I had asked God for forgiveness for everything that I could remember in my life. I was mentally, physically and spiritually drained from me trying to create life. It was time to visit a doctor to tell us the truth about what was happening. I found a doctor, based on a recommendation, and I immediately made an appointment. As soon as my husband and I were in his office, we were immediately disappointed. This man sat at his mahogany desk, with his crisp white jacket, the perfectly gelled hair, and the most beautiful blue eyes and said to me, "You need to lose up to 100 pounds." What the what? I only weighed 165 pounds at the time of this appointment. Yes, I had gained weight, but I had noticed other women a lot larger than I was and they were having babies back to back! That just told me that he was not interested in helping us start our family. I left saddened, but my husband encouraged me to seek a new doctor.

Fertility Specialist 2

A few weeks later, I found another fertility specialist, but we had to wait a month before getting an appointment with her. That month felt like the longest month ever. She *had* to be the real deal since she had a waitlist. Although I was excited, I experienced many emotions. I was ashamed that it had come to this to start our family. I kept the appointment between me and my husband.

4 PC WHAT? PCOS? WHAT THE HECK IS THAT?

Tears running down your face, and your heart's feeling like it's gonna break. And the earth feels like it's bout to shake. And you've taken all that you can take. Just remember where your help comes from. Realizing you got somewhere to run. Don't worry 'bout what you're going through. Instead of worrying, here's what you can do. Praise Him anyway. ~ **In the Middle, Isaac Carree**

We were finally able to see the doctor and after running bloodwork tests and performing an ultrasound, the physician sat in the patient room and informed us that I had polycystic ovarian syndrome/disease also known as PCOS/PCOD. Not only did she deliver the bad news of one disease, but she also told me that I was a Type 2 diabetic.

She may as well had given me my earth expiration date because it felt like she had stabbed me directly in my heart. I had never felt pains like that before. The entire time she talked to us, she was smiling. Why was she smiling? I was disappointed, hurt and confused.

PCOS and Diabetes at the same time?

I had never heard PCOS/PCOD nor did I have any idea what it was or what caused it. I only had a few questions for the doctor. What is this? How did I get this? What can you do to get rid of it? As she sat there talking about these new attacks on my body, I felt like I was having an outer body experience. I felt like I was going through the seven stages of grief, all at the same time. I felt like I was dying. I started to cry and tasted the saltiest tears I had ever tasted, maybe because there was so much hurt and heartbreak in those tears.

Shock was the first stage to hit me. I had just been diagnosed with some diseases about which I knew nothing. I would now have to take medicines to get rid of something that I didn't ask to enter my body. How did this happen? Was I being punished for something?

I was in total denial that this was possible. My regular OB/GYN had never mentioned anything to me about this! There's no way that this just happened. Did this doctor know what she was talking about?

Did they switch my results with another patient? I couldn't believe this! After trying to start our family for a whole year, I now had to put it on the backburner because I had to deal with these new issues.

I felt angry with the doctor for telling me! What was I supposed to do with this information? How was this going to factor in starting my family? I became angry at everybody, including myself. What had I done to my body to cause it to turn against me?

I felt that if I bargained with God, he would remove these illnesses from my body. I just needed to have my 1-on-1 talk with God. I knew He would never allow me to go through this by myself or right now when I desperately wanted to have children.

After not hearing a response from God through this doctor's mouth, not only was I angry, I was also saddened and depressed that it wasn't happening like I thought it should. Those salty tears just kept flowing with no end in sight. The room became blurry to me as I started to feel dizzy.

I began to grieve the children that I may never meet because I didn't know what PCOS or diabetes was doing or going to do to my body to prevent my heart's desire from being realized.

Even though the doctor had given such dire news, there was still a glimpse of hope that I would be that one in a million patient to prove her wrong. I believe that's when my faith was struggling to be my primary focus. I tried to understand and come to terms with what little I heard, but I was still a bit concerned about what it meant in starting a family.

To this day, I don't really remember too much about what the doctor said during that appointment. The only that I do remember is her saying that it may be harder to conceive. No joke! I'm grateful my husband was there to listen and get all the information I'd need later. I left that appointment feeling more depressed and far more confused. I felt more conflicted in more ways than I could explain.

Getting diagnosed with PCOS *and* diabetes only added to the grief that I had been enduring for the past couple of years.

My life had become a series of questions with no answers anywhere in sight. What was I supposed to do now? How was I supposed to start my family? How was I going to have my heart's desire of raising my own children and giving them all the love I had? God, why not me? Why can't I have children? Why would you create me so unperfect? I was having my very own pity party.

As quickly as I began to have hope that having children would happen for us, it quickly went away. I allowed sadness to creep in again. A week later, I decided to read the documents that the doctor provided. I wanted to know, for sure, what I was dealing with and what options were available to help. After reading the literature, I quickly realized that I was exhibiting all the signs and symptoms of this newly-diagnosed disease, PCOS.

The top five symptoms stopped me in my tracks. I've had irregular cycles my entire life. I remembered that my first ever cycle lasted 13 days! What teenage child should have that experience? Acne has been a bigger issue that it should be in my adult life.

Here I was scrubbing my face with witch hazel, alcohol and every other product on the market and nothing ever worked. Now things were starting to make some sense.

The most embarrassing thing is having hair grow in places where it shouldn't grow. Around 2005, I started noticing hair on my chin area. My sideburns were thick and long. Sometimes, I would see a shadow and would shave my upper lip area. I didn't know what was going on, but I knew I was not walking out of the house like that!

The next sign on the list was the inability to get pregnant. Wow! Now that I'm seeing this in black and white, with the other symptoms, it really started hitting home. The last symptom on the first page was weight gain. OMG! So, that's the reason for the 40-pound weight gain that I couldn't seem to lose!

There were many other symptoms of PCOS, like sleep apnea, depression, anxiety, abnormal uterine bleeding and endometrial cancer. Now, my mind started racing so fast that I became light-headed. I really didn't know what to make of all of this. I sat and just tried to take it all in. Even though I was able to read this, I still didn't know where it all started, and the doctor didn't have any definite answers.

After reading about the main signs and symptoms and how they all work against the body, I wanted to read the suggestions for helping to eliminate or reverse PCOS. The number one suggestion was to lose weight with lifestyle changes.

You have got to be kidding me! I've been trying to lose weight for years. It stated that if I was able to lose 5% of my body weight, it might help with this disease and could help increase the effectiveness of fertility medicines. Obviously, they didn't mean me because I tried for years and couldn't lose 1% of my weight.

I HAVE PCOS.

I AM OVERWEIGHT.

I HAVE ADULT ACNE.

I HAVE HIRSUTISM.

I HAVE TYPE 2 DIABETES.

Now I knew what had been causing me strife for a very long time. It was PCOS and all the complications that it brings to work against everything that I so desperately desired.

5 I'M GETTING MY BABY! BY ANY MEANS NECESSARY…

Even though your winds blow, I want you to know. You cause me no alarm cause I safe in His arms. Even though your rain falls, I can still make this call. Let there be peace. Now I can say go away, I command you to move today. Because of faith, I have a brand new day. The sun will shine, and I will be okay. That's what I told the storm! ~ I Told The Storm, Greg O'Quinn and Joyful Noize

After getting hit with the hard blow of PCOS, I spent the next 13 to 14 years trying every diet, purchasing every workout DVD, praying more, trying to find my internal peace, and becoming angrier because my plan wasn't working. No matter how many diets I tried, how many days I worked out or how intense the workouts were, I never saw any results.

If anything, I continued to gain weight. How was that even possible?! In 2001, I went from 150 pounds to 170 pounds.

I was now overweight, upset, frustrated and felt like quitting. The weight gain added another level of insecurity and self-consciousness. I felt like my body was fighting against me to be healthy. I was emotionally, mentally, and physically exhausted. I had never heard of anyone gaining weight while eating healthy *and* working out. Believe me, there was no increase in muscle, it was all unhealthy fat cells that somehow loved my midsection. In 2002, I gained another 15 pounds.

Every year after, I would gain an additional five to ten pounds. One year, I stopped gaining weight altogether. I had reached the golden weight of 237 pounds. When I would reveal my weight to others, they'd say that I didn't look like it. That made me feel good, to an extent. I still had to find a way to get this weight down.

Regardless of what my body was doing, I was set on having my baby, especially after he had been revealed to me in a beautiful dream. I remained hopeful that my baby boy would soon arrive. I knew I would have a son, I just didn't know when or how long I would have to wait.

The one thing that made it all hard and difficult was being asked by family members when were we planning on having children.

When are you all going to have children?

That question was hard to answer, and it was difficult to not think of the heartbreak that I was currently experiencing. I felt as if I was being judged because I didn't have any children. This just made me distance myself even more. I would meet other women and after they found out how long my husband and I had been married, they would ask the same question. My self-imposed distance from others only grew even more.

In 2007, I thought about other ways to start a family. I was fine with adopting a child or using a surrogate. So, I talked to my husband and we agreed to start the process of obtaining information about the adoption process. We thought it would be faster and less expensive. Boy, oh, boy, were we wrong!

Adoption Round 1

Not knowing the ins-and-outs of the adoption process, I went to work researching the best, easiest and fastest ways to adopt. I researched the requirements and disqualifications. The first choice was to adopt the kids that nobody seemed to want, which were the kids in foster care. We had stable jobs, no criminal records, and a big home that was ready to be filled with the sounds and laughter of children. This had to be the quickest and most straightforward way to start our family. So we thought!

After contacting the local child services agency, we were told informed that a number of things would be needed, to include attending a training session for two weekends, prior to us being allowed to meet the children or adopt them. They were very direct by telling me that both my husband and I must attend all training sessions, or we would not be able to complete the process. We agreed.

Each day, we arrived, signed in and took our normal seats to get that day's training. It was a lot of information to take in, but we were ready for any challenges that would come our way. We were finally going to start our family!

After the training, the process became stagnant. I would call to check on the process and would be met with the message that they'd be in contact with us soon. "Well, what's soon?", I asked. It's been a month already! It felt like they weren't really interested in finding homes for those beautiful, innocent children. I became so frustrated with waiting that I asked one of the social workers if they did this for job security. I asked, "Is it part of the process to get families interested and then make them wait so long that they lose interest?" The response was always the same. "We're working your case now." I'm sure this caused even more delays.

What's Really Going On?

Our assigned social worker finally reached out to us three weeks later to advise us that we needed to complete the questionnaire that she was mailing to us, and then we'd need to schedule our home visits with her. At this same time, she also advised that she was totally booked with home visits for the next two months and we would be put on her waiting list. After receiving and completing the form and having our fingerprints submitted, we received one excuse after another for why we still had to wait. The first lie, um, excuse, was that we both didn't attend all days of the training sessions. Wait, what? That's not true because I made sure that we both signed all the sheets.

The next excuse was that they claimed to have never received our questionnaire that took us hours to fill in. Ridiculous! Lucky for her, I had a copy and was able to drive to her and place it in her hands. Needless to say, she was not very enthused by this action. Even with being met with such resistance, I was willing to deal with it and I felt it was worth it if we could just get our children.

We sat and waited for a call to schedule our home study visits. That call never came. My calls and voicemails went unanswered. I was becoming more and more frustrated and confused with this nonsense. I searched and found a social worker that could do our homestudy and hired her. She came in and completed the three required homestudies and we contacted the agency to advise them that we no longer needed a home study. Again, they weren't happy with this action.

Later, we were finally able to identify children to whom we felt we could be great parents. We even identified a sibling set of three that we felt should remain together and wanted them in our home. The social worker advised that the children were available for adoption and she would review our home study to see if we were good candidates.

A week later, she called and left a voicemail stating that none of the children were available anymore. Now, she was really playing with my emotions! Why would they do something like this? God, why is this happening to me? Did you not create me to be a mother? Why would you give me all of this love to share, but no one with whom to share it? I was consumed with this frustration and hurt for a month or two until I came up with my next grand plan.

Adoption Round 2

We're going to work with a private agency! I know since they want to get paid, they are going to deliver a baby. I really didn't know how messed up the adoption world really was. After researching several private adoption agencies, I was in sticker shock!

Why would they charge so much when the parents would need that money to care for the child? I sought to contact the best agencies that offered reasonable costs and received their literature by mail. I then narrowed it down to two agencies that specialized in African-American adoptions. I thought it would go even faster, based on the research that I'd done.

After filling out the paperwork for each agency, I had to take a step back. Something at home was feeling a bit off. I didn't feel that my husband was still as enthused as he once was. I then realized that I hadn't taken the time to ask him how he was doing. I had never stopped to allow him the time to be as vocal as he needed to be. I was just consumed with having our home filled with children. My husband and I sat and talked about the adoption process, and that conversation ended in heartbreak.

He told me that he was no longer interested in adopting.

I'm not really interested in adopting anymore.

Now, what am I supposed to do? Why would he let me do all that I've been doing if he really wasn't on board? I felt like my life had just ended. I thought he wanted this just as much as I did! I was in a silent stage of frustration, aggravation, denial, fury, heartbrokenness, and confusion. I didn't know what to think or how to think. After a whole year of trying to adopt and now realizing it wasn't going to happen, I was all out of ideas.

I remained disappointed with my husband for quite some time and would often find myself questioning his motives on many other things. I also didn't invest in too many projects that required him to be on board. I didn't know if he would continue do that with everything else.

I gave up!

I decided to give up. If I couldn't have my own children, I would just do things for other people's children to see a smile on their faces. I became a Godmother and absolutely loved it. Even though it was long distance, I received plenty of pictures and was able to hear her sweet little voice on the phone all the time. I love my Mary! I was ok with this lifestyle. I began thinking about other things that I wanted to do in life and I made myself busy with every kind of arts and crafts activity that I could think to do. I started being OK with working longer hours to get tasks done, sometimes being the last one in the office. I just didn't want to go home and do nothing.

In 2009, we did a major family move to Georgia to assist with a family medical condition. With the activity surrounding us in dealing with the situation, I didn't have the time, nor the energy to focus on what I didn't have. I became busy praying for healing and recovery for our ill family member. I felt that he needed blessings from God more than I did. During this time, I had someone tell me that I had a pure spirit and a good heart. They admired how I was so selfless and thought of others before my own desires. I responded, stating that's how we all should be in life. If we can put others first and go to God on their behalf, that is pleasing to God and He is only one I live to please. When you willingly do for others, God will bless you more abundantly than you could ever pray to receive.

In 2010, and after getting settled in the new state, I secured a new job and met a new friend who just happened to have a 2-year-old. We had a natural click and our friendship began. I tried my best to stay busy. Even though I wasn't seeing a doctor, silently I was hoping that I would get pregnant, naturally. I tried my best to stay busy, not allowing myself to think about what I really wanted, and it became easier to continue focusing on others.

Fertility Specialist 3

In late 2010, I found a fertility specialist who told us that, based on our test results, there was no reason that we shouldn't already have children. I felt the same way! We decided to do a timed cycle to see if that would work. If nothing happened, we would then move on to medically-advanced options.

By 2011, it was time to make another family move. This time we moved to Massachusetts. That meant that we weren't able to go back to the same doctor in Georgia to start other fertility options, but I was OK with it because we were now in an area where I'd heard about some great fertility doctors. I took some time to learn the landscape since I knew we'd be there for a while. After getting comfortable with the area and people, I did my research, read reviews and, in early 2012, I made an appointment with the fertility doctor that was first available.

Fertility Specialist 4

This new doctor ran more tests on both me and my husband. After reviewing the results, this doctor also seemed baffled about why we didn't have any children yet. The one question that each doctor always asked was "Have you ever been pregnant?" To me, that was the most ridiculous question ever. I was at the appointment for them to help me get pregnant!

Have you ever been pregnant?

Even though I was truly frustrated with the line of questioning, we decided to move forward with a process called IUI or Intrauterine Insemination. We were now using technology and not just pills, tests and timing. This had to work! No one told me the range of emotions I would experience from the number of medicines, excitement, nervousness, and disbelief. The closer it got to the insemination day, the more my nerves were going haywire. I didn't know how to feel; I just wanted it to happen NOW!

For two weeks, we waited before going back to confirm pregnancy. We arrived at the clinic, had bloodwork taken and met with the doctor, who advised us that it didn't happen this time. Again, we were not pregnant. I just cried. I felt like I had gone through all of this for nothing.

What happened? What didn't the doctor do to ensure that I would be pregnant? Why couldn't this happen for us, even with technology on our side? I was at a loss for words.

I was now upset, hurt, and disappointed all over again. Not only was I emotionally and spiritually hurting, but after visiting so many different doctors over the years, I was beginning to feel the financial burden of it all. After getting to the acceptance that it didn't happen this time, I still longed for a child, so we decided to try again. Still, no success. At one point, I felt as if I was intentionally torturing myself.

We made a final family move in 2013, and I was back at it again. I checked in to adoption information, even though my husband had previously stated that he was no longer open to the idea of adoption. I also researched local fertility specialists and did research on the best and the most cost-effective since I may need to have multiple procedures performed to get pregnant. I was very determined to start our family. I was tired of being heartbroken over something that seemed to come so easily to others. I could feel and see my biological clock ticking. It was time to make this happen.

Fertility Specialist 5

In late 2014, I scheduled an appointment with a fertility center and the doctor suggested a timed cycle and then an IUI. Even though I knew in my heart that it was not going to work, we went ahead with the procedure.

During those 60 days, I felt like a number more than a person or patient. I didn't feel like I received the one-on-one attention that I had with other doctors. I felt that perhaps that was the way it was done in this new area. I just wanted my baby by any means necessary! It turned out to be another two months of unsuccessful trying.

By now, you'd think that I'd be accustomed to the disappointment. Absolutely not! I knew it was coming, but there was no way to really prepare for it. I remained hopeful about it all, but my heart still ached.

My heart ached.

I decided to put more fertility specialists on hold for a while and investigated the adoption process again. I thought it would be a different experience in a place that's more progressive. Unfortunately, it was not. I dealt with some of the same foolishness as I had before.

It made me feel like the social workers really didn't want the kids to be adopted. With so much abuse happening to kids in the foster system, I felt like they weren't interested in doing their jobs either. Yes, I was back to my judgmental stage.

Adoption Round 3

Instead of playing around and wasting time on the state's adoption process, I decided to research private adoptions again. I wasn't really concerned about my husband not being interested, I knew he would come around. I knew he wanted children just as much as I wanted them. We would, at times, talk about how our children would be ~ the personalities, looks and quirks. Those were great and funny conversations, but I was tired of talking about them. I was ready to see and hold my children.

I reviewed so many different adoption agency websites until I was oftentimes confused about which agency offered what services. That was leading into 2015.

After speaking to a few of the agencies, I decided that there was just so much red tape, and I just didn't have the energy to try to cut through the first layer of it.

I left adoption alone altogether, but I knew I wasn't done trying. Even after all the heartache that I'd been through since 1999, I still had some fight left in me. I heard this saying that "If you want something in life, you have to work hard for it." That used to be one of the sayings that I lived by, even though it was the total opposite of my real beliefs. I truly believed and still believe that if what you want in life is meant for you, it'll come to you as easy as you asked for it, in God's time. We must be patient and trust in His promise.

Fertility Specialist 6

In March 2015, I told my husband that I wanted to give it one more try. He agreed, and I located a new fertility center that offered IVF. I was lucky to find one that offered a discount for military families. This **had** to be a sign from God! We made the appointment, had bloodwork testing, and answered the same questions that I'd been asked a million times before. After that was all done, it was time to start the process.

I was put on the multiple required medicines, which had the worst mental and emotional effects on me. My emotions were all over the place. I would cry for nothing at all. I cried opening the mail and reading about an auto financial offer. What was I crying for, I hadn't applied for a car loan?! Injecting those hormones into my body made me feel like I was losing my mind! Anything to get my baby.

The day finally arrived for the egg retrieval. We went in and came out a few hours later and were told that they were able to retrieve a total of nine eggs. WooHoo! We were excited, but had to now wait for the technician to inseminate the eggs and watch them grow.

The fertilized eggs were to be placed in my uterus on Day 3, but we received a call to say they would wait until Day 4 or Day 5 to give the eggs more time to grow. On the day of embryo transfer, we were told that only one egg was of good quality and one more egg was ok for transfer. The rest didn't take the fertilization process.

I was shocked, but also excited to know that I would be pregnant as soon as they inserted my eggs and they attached to the uterus. The dreaded two-week waiting period had to happen and then I'd go back for a blood test to confirm pregnancy. This had to work! Those two weeks passed by so slowly. I did nothing, but move at a snail's pace and sat for the entire two weeks to make sure I didn't do anything to jeopardize my eggs from attaching to my uterus.

At the two-week mark, I stopped by the doctor's office for my blood test on my way to work and was advised that I would receive a call by the afternoon with the results. I was excited and wore a smile all day, even though no one at work knew why I was smiling. I called and informed my husband know that I had made it to work and would let him know the result once I received it. We were excited!

Around 2 pm, I received the call I had been waiting for two weeks to receive! It was the fertility clinic. The nurse called to advise me that I was not pregnant. I was totally heartbroken! I felt so alone. I felt like I going to die. I felt my heart actually breaking.

Dear, you are not pregnant.

I didn't how else to feel and, since I hadn't told anyone about this process, I didn't know who to call or what to say. I left my office and went to the restroom, to try and compose myself. I called my husband and he tried to calm me down. It didn't help. He offered to come and pick me up, but I told him no and that I needed to keep busy.

I didn't want to leave early and have people trying to figure out what was wrong with me. I just didn't want to talk to anyone.

I stayed in the bathroom and just talked to God for about ten minutes. I cried and cried, still talking to God to help me get it together. I was so distraught and felt like I would stop breathing at any moment. Why didn't I tell them to call my husband? Why did I think this would really work? I felt like I had set myself up for the biggest failure to date.

This was my last-ditch effort of trying to create a new life. I was now starting to realize that it would never happen for us. We weren't created to be parents, at least not together. If it hadn't happened over the past 16 years, it wasn't going to happen now. I had to get to this way of thinking and get there fast if I was going to be able to move forward.

There was no way that I would inject myself with any more hormones from any process that seemed to cause more harm than good. There was no way that I could allow myself to keep going on this self-induced destructive track of life. There was no way that I could allow myself to become even more depressed, saddened or heartbroken.

I was done with trying to create life. I was done with trying to make plans on how things would happen. I was done with everything. I Was Done!

I Was Done.

By June 2015, I decided to move forward with my application to become a Big Sister with the Big Brother Big Sister Organization. I felt that if God hadn't created me to be a mother, I knew that He blessed me to be a great Big Sister. I had an awesome track record! I was quickly matched with my Little Sister Ashanti. It was the perfect match! We ended up having quite a few things in common. She is smart, outgoing, determined and ready to tackle the world. My kind of girl! Truthfully, I needed her and her youthful energy.

Being able to be in the presence of this young lady brightened my day when my days were full of clouds and gloom. I knew that she would rely on me being the best version of myself; therefore, I had to make sure that I had myself together for all of the activities that we would do every weekend. I had fun and I know she had fun too.

Watching her blossom and turn into the best version of herself kept me motivated to do the right thing and being the role model that I signed up to be. Our constant contact helped me get over thinking of myself and all that didn't go right. I was able to see greatness in her and pour my love and big sister advice into her life. She continued to amaze me every single day. I felt blessed.

6 LETTING GO

As soon as I stopped worrying. Worrying how the story ends. I let go and I let God. Let God have His way. That's when things started happening. When I stopped looking at back then. I let go and I let God. Let God have His way. ~ Let Go, Dewayne Woods

The fresh start of 2016 was a great thing for me. With all that I had been through over the last 17 years, I was ready to do something different. I pulled out my notebook binder and reviewed the tabbed sections for everything that I wanted to accomplish in this life. There was a total of seven sections, but I had only named four of them ~ a women's clothing store, a kids' clothing store, an adult store for couples and writing a children's book series.

After a quick review, I had to think through each to see which would be the easiest and fastest to implement. That's when the project management side of my brain kicked in, and I planned each event out through the grand opening.

I decided to start with the women's clothing store that I named Silhouettes. This was in January 2016 and I had planned the grand opening for April 2016, not leaving a lot of time. With only three months to implement my plan, I had a lot of work to do, including registering my store's name with the state and local authorities, finding a physical store location, researching wholesale options, and purchasing store equipment. I had to work on my marketing plan and think of hiring someone to work during the weekdays. It was a lot to do, but I had nothing but time on my hands.

April 2016 arrived, and it was a success! My store was open, the website was up and running, and I was ready for business. I stayed busy making sure to stay ahead of the current trends at the most affordable prices. May and June 2016 produced successful online sales. There was more traffic online than at the physical store, so I decided to venture out and become a fashion vendor at different events to get more awareness about the physical store location. Another great successful business decision!

July 2016 was a different month. I felt something that kept pulling on my spirit. Toward the end of July, I sat in my home office and started my daily conversation with God. I talked to Him about things that were going on in my life, what I had planned to do with the store. I asked him for a sign that I was planning was the right move. I would also always pray for His blessing over my household, spirit, and business, as well as, over my family and friends.

After that talk, I still felt the tugging on my spirit. I started talking to God again, but this time, instead of telling Him of my upcoming plans, I started apologizing.

I started apologizing for everything that I could remember that I may have done that wasn't right in His eyes. I apologized for getting an attitude with my husband for taking my *last* cookie. I apologized for ignoring my husband when I heard him calling my name when I knew he *really* didn't want anything. I apologized for everything! I finally arrived at the biggest apology that I think He was waiting for me to do. I apologized to God for trying to do His job ~ create life.

I knew better. I was raised to know that God is everything and the only Creator of life. I was taught that if there was something that I wanted, I should pray about it, put it in God's hands and have the faith that He would bless me in His timing.

It finally hit me that, after all these years, I had been trying to do what only God can do. Once I apologized, I felt an immediate release of all the hurt, disappointment, sadness, depression, and failures that had been buried. That release also released tears of joy because I finally felt free to fully walk in my faith without feeling held back by my spirit. I knew that I had just done what God desired for me to do. I was now totally free to live my life the way He intended.

In August 2016, I attended another vending event, but almost canceled because I wasn't feeling well. I was encouraged by Tasha, who was my retail stylist, to just go since I had already paid. She and I went forward, and I was glad that I did.

We had an awesome time and it turned out to be one of the best and most profitable events that we had attended. By late August, I could tell that my body was telling me to slow down.

I knew that I had been on-the-go for the first half of the year with my store and my professional career. Now my body was giving me the signs that I needed to rest. I began to get nauseous and experience occasional dizzy spells. So, I took a few days off to let my body rest. A few days later, while talking to a co-worker who knew my fertility struggles over the past 17 years, she asked me to take a pregnancy test. I thought she had lost her mind, but I knew she was coming from a sincere place. Even though I wasn't really interested in going back to that once hurtful place or time in my past, I told her that I would get one and let her know when it came back negative.

Being true to my word, I called my husband and asked him to stop by the pharmacy to pick up a digital pregnancy test. Of course, he now had a ton of questions. I could only laugh as I imagined his facial expressions as the thoughts raced through his mind. When he returned home, he gave me the bag that contained the tests. These were the tests that had one line for negative and two lines for positive, exactly what I didn't ask him to purchase. I asked him why didn't he purchase the digital test that I asked him to purchase. His response, "I forgot."

In my head, I was thinking "don't send a man to do a woman's job!"

*Never send a man
to do a woman's job!*

I had used these tests so many times that I was already prepared for what it would show. I went ahead and used the first one and after a few minutes, it showed two lines. I disregarded it and told my husband that it must be a defective one. He asked that I use the second one in a couple of hours. I did, and it also showed two lines. Again, I disregarded it and told him that I'd like to go get a digital test to use in the morning.

We returned to the pharmacy and I purchased a digital test. The next morning, I tested, and it showed in big letters YES+. I was shocked, floored, confused, speechless and thrilled, all at the same time! After surprising my husband out of his morning sleep to tell him the news, we were both excited that we were finally pregnant. Neither of us could think back to when conception would have happened. I had to wait until Monday, 2 days away, to call and make an appointment to confirm and find out how far along we were in the pregnancy. We arrived at the appointment on Tuesday, still unsure that this was even real until we saw the heartbeat. We were told that we were six weeks into the pregnancy.

All I could do was cry at how gracious, wonderful and marvelous God truly is. He will always keep His word to us. He is all that and a bag of chips! (*Funyuns, to be exact…lol*)

I remember crying so much and still in shock from it all. I just wanted to sit in the corner and hold my belly that was nurturing the life that God had so easily created. I knew he would be the perfect little boy. He would be the best little boy on this side of Earth. Yes, I already knew the baby would be a boy.

God had already revealed him to me. Plus, I had spent the last 15 years shopping for girl's and boy's clothes and had given away all of the girl's clothing to a friend for a baby shower gift. With only boy's clothing left, there was no way God would give me a daughter at this time. My husband and I were so elated and would often talk about what our future son would be like, his personality and possible likes and dislikes. It was a fun pregnancy on most days, but that was probably because I was so excited about this new life that I didn't remember my morning sickness experience.

We were finally pregnant, and it seemed to easily happen for us now that I didn't feel the need to do God's job. I stopped thinking about all that I had gone through trying to get to this point and started thanking God for all of his great blessings, big and small.

I continued to thank God for everything each and every day. During the next eight months of pregnancy, it allowed me the time to continue restoring my faith in God for everything. My relationship with God became so great that if I asked for something, it would be revealed to me as soon as I asked.

I was and still am in awe of God's blessings and my relationship with Him.

Also, during this time, we set up the nursery, and I was able to do all my arts and crafts projects and we decorated his room even more. I was proud of what we were able to create for our little blessed bundle of joy. We decided on a name, even though it was a name that I had chosen ten years earlier. His name would be Aspen Baylor and he would be born in April 2017.

7 LIFE LESSONS

I've got a vision and a purpose. A divine destiny. It may not look like it right now, but faith ain't what I see. It is the thing I hope for, believing it will come. And no matter how long it takes, I know God's will shall be done. ~ Destiny, Tina Campbell

There are many lessons that I've learned and re-learned during these past 18 years of trying to start my family. To sum it up, here are a few that I still use every single day.

God is God alone. He can do what no one else can. There will be many that will try to imitate God. You can imitate man, but God is not a regular man. He is God Almighty, our Creator. There is nothing that you think you can do that God can't do at a greater level.

God's timing is not my timing. When I ask God for something, I had to know that He may not come when I want Him, but He will always come right on time.

All you have to do is try Him. He will never let you down. You must believe in Him. There were many times where I felt like I had to do it. I felt like the one step that I was doing wasn't enough. I needed to make more steps before God's blessing would kick in. That's not true at all. All I had to do was try Jesus and believe in His blessings over my life.

Put it in God's hands and leave it there. I learned this lesson at a very young age, but it wasn't until I was older that I actually understood the meaning behind this saying. To me, this means that I shouldn't be stressing over things nor still trying to work on things when I say that I'm putting it in God's hands. When I put it in God's hands, I have to totally let it go and let God do His thing, in His timing.

If you have faith the size of a mustard seed; anything is possible. I read this in the bible a long time ago, and again, it wasn't until I got older that I really knew what this meant. Now, I can see that my faith has been fully restored in God and His marvelous works. I don't worry about anything. I don't stress over the little things in life. I just thank God in advance for fixing whatever needs to be fixed in my life, personally, spiritually, mentally, financially and emotionally.

8 MY PRAYER FOR YOU

Now I know there were days I looked at myself, I felt like less of a person compared to everyone else. What about this flaw, too big, too small, can I exchange? And trying to make up for where I fell short, I let sense slip away. And when I look in the mirror and don't look like what I see. Oh, I just thank you for always lovin' me. And I know I get bad but you wait patiently. I just want to thank you for always lovin' me. ~ Lovin' Me, Jonathan McReynolds

Dear God,

I pray that you allow the people reading this book to fall so deeply in love with you and who You are. I pray that they become so wrapped up in serving you that they can't look to the world for things that only You can provide. I pray for their beautiful lives and that you bless them so abundantly with every one of their heart's desires.

I pray that you allow them to know that if they only believe in You, they will live a more abundant, happy, enriched and fulfilled life.

I pray for their mental, spiritual, financial, physical and emotional health right now. I pray that whatever is broken in them, that you heal it and mend it so that it appears as if it were never broken. Because that's the kind of God that You are.

I pray that you allow this book of my journey to serve as a witness to your greatness when the world throws things to make them stumble. You are a mountain mover; allow them to come to you and believe that you will provide them with the strength to climb over any mountain.

Lord, I pray that you make every enemy that arises against them, make them a footstool. You said ask and ye shall receive, so I'm asking that you bless all the people that read this book. Bless them with the knowledge that as long as they are living for you, you will continually bless them and their lives.

And Jesus said unto them, Because of your unbelief: for verily I say unto you, If ye have faith as a grain of mustard seed, ye shall say unto this mountain, Remove hence to yonder place; and it shall remove; and nothing shall be impossible unto you.

Matthew 17:20 Bible, King James Version

If You have blessed me, I know You can do it for anyone else. In Jesus' name, I pray. Amen.

ABOUT THE AUTHOR

Tameka Chapman is a high achiever and highly regarded transformational speaker. She has the ability to get her audience to see and feel the story throughout her presentations. This once spiritually, mentally and financially broken woman has been made whole by restoring her faith in God, His timing and His way. For her belief and restored faith, she has been abundantly blessed and made whole in all areas of her brokenness.

Tameka is a current resident of Northern Virginia where she resides with her husband Deone and their handsome son, Aspen. She is a transformational speaker, girls mentor, author, and a singer. She is also the creator of the *Torn, Mended, now Healed* Women's Empowerment Seminars, helping to heal women by showing them the path to restoring their faith. During her downtime, she loves family road trips, playing with her son, reading, and solving sudoku puzzles.

You can reach Tameka at the following contact information:

Facebook – Twitter – Instagram   @TamekaEmpowers

Email: TamekaEmpowers@yahoo.com

Website: TamekaEmpowers.com